CPAN, CAPA

Study Guide for Postanesthesia and Perianestesia Nurses

Tori Marsh MSN, RN, CNOR

Copyright © 2021
Tori Marsh
All rights reserved

Contents

Introduction 4
Recommended Reading 6
Glossary 8
Test Knowledge 10
Phases of care 11
Patient Care 13
    Legal forms and Orders 13
    NPO guidelines: 14
    Culture of Safety 15
    Normal vital signs 16
    Normal lab values 19
Sedation and Nerve Blocks 20
    OSA- 23
Scoring tools 25
Emergency Situations 28
    Malignant Hyperthermia- 28
    Blood transfusion reaction 29
Special Patient Considerations 30
    Pregnancy 30
    The Elderly 30
    Infants and children 31
Medications 32
CAPA Example Questions 36
CAPA Example Questions Answers and Rationales 44
CPAN Example Questions 47
CPAN Example Questions Answers and Rationales 55
CPAN/CAPA Example Questions 58
CPAN/CAPA Example Questions Answers and Rationales 74
CAPA/ CPAN Crossword Puzzle 81
Blank Note Pages 90

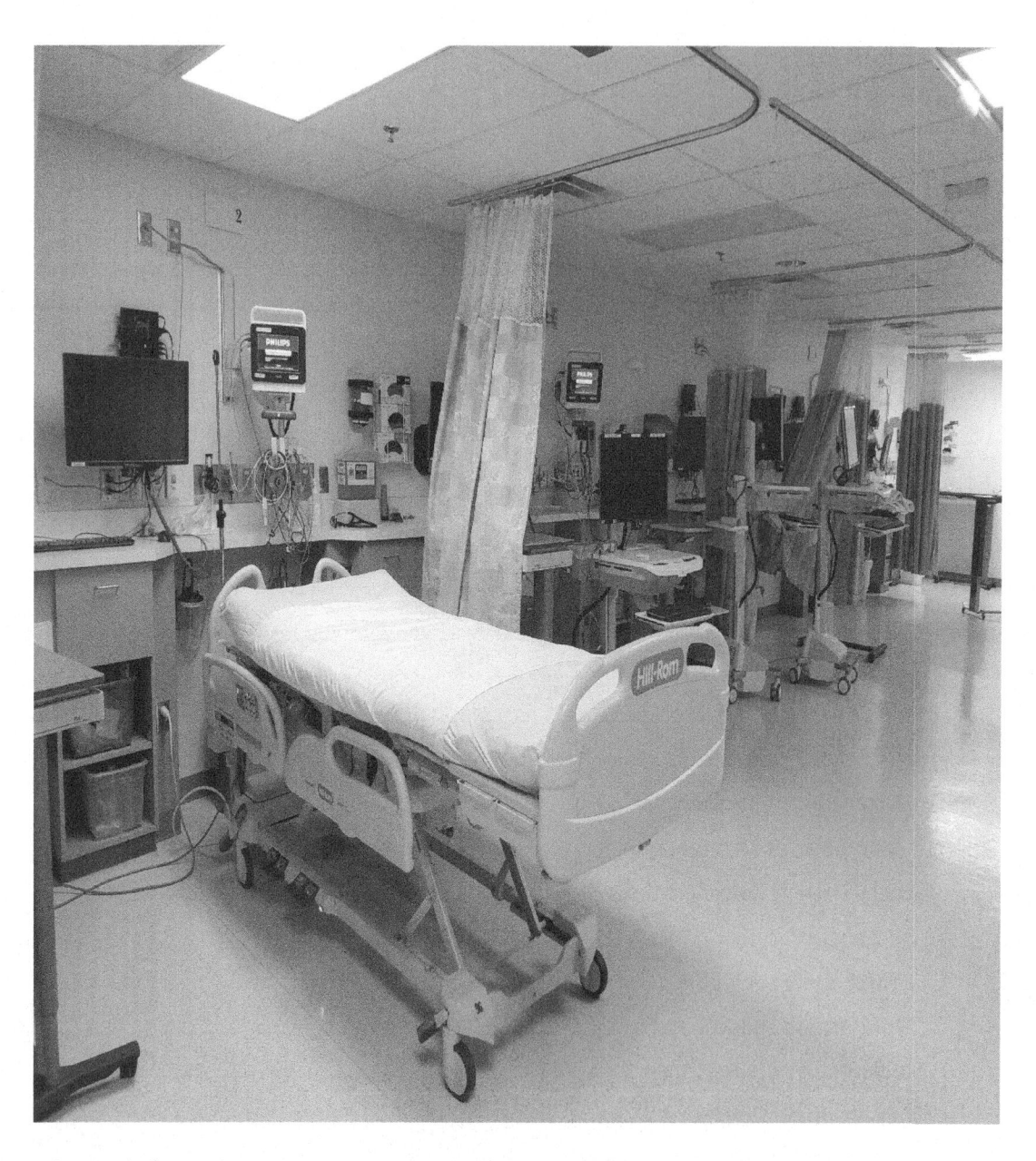

A PACU ready for patients.

Introduction

The Certified Post Anesthesia Nurse certification, CPAN, is a certification for nurses who work in post anesthesia care. These nurses practice in the PACU or recovery room, which is considered a critical care area. To be eligible to sit for the exam, a nurse must have at least 1200 hours of experience in this area.

The CAPA certification, which stands for Certified Ambulatory Perianesthesia nurse, is a certification for those nurses who practice in the pre-operative and phase two recovery areas. These nurses need 1200 hours experience in these areas.

Many healthcare settings combine pre-op, phase 1 and phase 2 care areas. Some settings combine phase 1 and phase 2. It is not uncommon for nurses to become certified for both the CAPA and the CPAN. This study guide was written for the nurse who wishes to become certified as both CAPA and CPAN.

If you only plan to sit for one of the exams, this book will help you as well. There are many questions on the CPAN exam that may also be seen on the CAPA and vice versa. Taking practice exams have been shown to help prepare for the actual test conditions and can help reduce anxiety.

When you decide that you want to become certified, your next step is to decide which test to take. If you have enough practice hours for both tests, and feel confident in your knowledge base, you can sit for both. There are several factors to consider when deciding on which test to take or if you want to take both. Cost is a factor. Will you be paying for the tests and testing materials on your own or will your employer help with the costs? Will you get a raise or another financial incentive if you are certified? Will you get more if you have two certifications? Are either of the certifications required for your job? Do you feel your knowledge base is stronger in one area over another?

To help decide which test to take go to cpancapa.org. All the information about the testing is located there. On the website you will also find practice questions and test day information. Read the handbook online carefully, there is a lot of information.

You decided on what certification(s) you want, congratulations! You have read the handbook and all information on cpancapa.org and are ready to schedule the test. Ask your employer if there is any financial assistance available. Ask your co-workers if they have any study materials or any advice on the test. Look over the information and decide how much study time you need. Sign up for the test, hopefully two or three months from now. Make a study plan. Use the blueprint online to help you. Research any procedures not commonly done at your facility that you may not be familiar with. If any co-workers or nurse friends are taking the same exam as you, decide if a study group would benefit you.

Find out where the testing center is. The testing center may not be in your town. The day of the test is not the time to get lost searching through a strange place. Try and get a good night's sleep. Don't laugh, it can happen even for nurses. Wear comfortable clothes to the testing center. They take security very seriously. You will be given a locker to put all your belongings in. You will be asked to turn out your pockets and roll down your socks. You will be wanded by a metal detector.

During the test, try and read the question and think of the answer in your head before looking at the given answers. If the answer in your head matches one given, go with it. Do not second guess yourself. If you do not know the answer, read all choices. If still struggling, answers involving safety are usually a good bet. Sometimes the longer answers are also right. Avoid answers that use words such as always or never. Healthcare is usually not absolute.

This book was designed to be written in. Use it to take notes, highlight anything you want to look at later or cross out what you already know. Use this book however it benefits you. There are several sections in the book to help with your study schedule. There is a section on test knowledge to help remind you of topics that you should know that may be on the test. There are sections with example questions to test your knowledge and to help you practice for taking the exam. There are blank pages for you to write in your own notes. There is even a crossword puzzle if you like those.

Good luck! You got this!

Recommended Reading

Cpancapa.org. *Certification Candidate Handbook.*

American Society of PeriAnesthesia Nurses (2019-2020). *Perianesthesia Nursing Standards Practice Recommendations and Interpretive Statements.* New Jersey, ASPAN.

American Heart Association. *ACLS Provider Manual.* Use the most current edition.

American Heart Association. *PALS Provider Manual.* Use the most current edition.

Marsh, T. (2021). *The Certified Ambulatory Perianesthesia Nurse CAPA Study Guide.*

Marsh, T. (2021). *Certified Postanesthesia Nurse CPAN Study Guide.*

Odom-Forren, J. (2018). *Drain's Perianesthesia Nursing, A Critical Care Approach.* St. Louis, Missouri, Elsevier.

Schick, L., Windle, P. (2021). *Perianesthesia Nursing Core Curriculum: Preprocedure, Phase 1 and Phase 2 PACU Nursing.* St. Louis, Missouri, Elsevier.

Glossary

- ACLS- Advanced Cardiac Life Support. You will see questions pertaining to this topic on the test. Most hospitals require phase one nurses to have their ACLS certification.

- ASPAN- The American Society of PeriAnesthesia Nurses.

- ASU- Ambulatory Surgery Unit.

- Beneficence- Helping others, doing good.

- CAM- Complementary and alternative medicines. - CAT- Complementary and alternative treatments.

- CA-UTI- Catheter associated urinary tract infection.

- Chvostek's sign- Positive if when cheeks are tapped over facial nerve, the facial muscles twitch. Indicates low calcium levels which can cause nerve excitability.

- Chlorhexidine gluconate- topical antibacterial, anti-infective agent. Used in surgical skin prep. Skin prep can be dyed orange or blue to easily see what skin areas have been prepped.

- CLA-BSI-Central line associated bloodstream infection.

- CRNA- Certified Registered Nurse Anesthetist.

- HIPPA- Health Insurance Portability and Accountability Act.

- MDROs- Multidrug-resistant organisms.

- Negative pressure isolation rooms- A room with lower pressure than adjacent rooms which prevents air from flowing out.

- Negligence- When a nurse fails to do what a similar situated, reasonable, and prudent professional would have done in similar circumstances.

- Never events- Preventable errors that the hospital will not be reimbursed for by Medicare. Retained objects from surgery, pressure ulcers, surgical site infections, catheter-associated infections and others are in this category.

- Nonmaleficence- Do no harm.

- OSA- Obstructive Sleep Apnea

- PACU- Posta Anesthesia Care Unit

- PALS- Pediatric Advanced Life Support. Nurses who recover children are often required to hold PALS certification.

- Postural hypotension- When a patient's blood pressure falls more than 20% from sitting to standing.

- PONV- Post-Op Nausea and Vomiting

- Pulse pressure- the difference between the systolic and diastolic blood pressure.

- R.A.C.E- What to do in a fire- Rescue, Activate alarm, Contain the fire, Evacuate/ Extinguish.

- RICE- Rest, ICE, Compression, Elevation.

- Root cause analysis- Investigation into sentinel events to address what can be done to prevent the occurrence in the future.

- Sentinel event- Incidents involving death or risk of serious injury. These events indicate a need for investigation into the cause to prevent a recurrence in the future.

- Stir up regimen- Deep breathing, coughing, position, mobilization, pain relief.

- Tort law- An act or omission that causes injury or harm. Medical malpractice is a subset of this. A retained surgical item will fall under this category.

- Transducer- A device for converting one form of energy into another. The transducer on CVP and arterial blood pressure monitors converts pressure energy into electrical energy that the monitor can process.

- Universal protocol- Required by the Joint Commission. Used to increase safety. Includes marking the surgical site, time-outs, pre-op verification process.

- Universal precautions- Treating all individuals as though they have contaminated body fluids. Emphasis on needle stick precautions.

- VRE- Vancomycin-resistant enterococcus

Test Knowledge

The information in this book follows the testing blueprint and may include information you will need to know for the exam. The three main topics are physiological needs, behavioral health and cognitive needs, and safety. These topics make up a percentage of the test as follows:

CPAN-Certified Post Anesthesia nurse
    Physiological needs 57%
    Behavioral health and cognitive needs 18%
    Safety 25%

CAPA- Certified Ambulatory Perianesthesia nurse
    Physiological needs 50%
    Behavioral health and cognitive needs 21%
    Safety 29%

Read the information on the website Cpancapa.org to make sure these numbers have not changed since the printing of this book. The testing blueprint is also available online. Review the blueprints to assess your strengths and opportunities to improve, to help guide your study plan.

Phases of care

- Preanesthesia phase. This area is focused on preparation for surgery. This is the pre op area. Assessment of the patients physical, mental, and spiritual needs is completed to identify issues needing to be addressed. If this phase is completed the day of surgery, the nursing care may also include education on what to expect in the following phases of care and possibly discharge teaching. When nurses are proficient in this area of nursing, they demonstrate their knowledge by taking the CAPA exam.

    - Staffing for Preanesthesia depends on the patient acuity, age of patients and if needed, sedation for preoperative nerve blocks. If a nurse is caring for a patient receiving conscious sedation, that nurse should have no other responsibilities.

- Postanesthesia phase 1. This is the immediate post-operative area. This is the PACU or recovery room. The patient may need assistance with breathing or other life saving measures. The patient requires constant attention. Nurses who are proficient in this area can take the CPAN exam.

    - Staffing for phase 1 post anesthesia care should be one nurse to one patient or one nurse to two patients. New admissions to the unit should be closely monitored until critical needs are met, such as airway and vital signs are stable, the initial assessment is completed, and the patient is calm, without combativeness or agitation.

    - There should be at least two nurses in the unit, one who is caring for the patient and one who is immediately available to provide assistance as needed. One nurse in the unit must be competent in phase 1 nursing care.

    - The nurse may have two patients if both are hemodynamically stable, conscious, over age eight, or, under age eight with a family or caregiver at bedside.

    - The nurse may have one patient if under 8 years old and unconscious.

    - The nurse may have one patient who is not conscious but hemodynamically stable, with a stable airway over the age of eight and one patient who is conscious and stable.

    - Occasionally one patient who is critical and unstable, may require two nurses.

- Postanesthesia phase 2. The patients in this area are preparing to go home. This is the area where the patient receives discharge instructions. The patient still requires monitoring for complications related to surgery or medications. Nurses with this specialty can sit for the CAPA certification.

    - Staffing for phase 2 should be one nurse to up to three patients. Staffing decisions should be made based on patient safety.

    - The nurse can care for three patients if over the age of eight or under age eight with family present.

    - If the patient is under age eight without family or support staff, the nurse-to-patient ratio should be one nurse to two patients.

    - Two staff members are required to be in the unit at all times. One must be an RN competent in phase 2 nursing.

    - Staffing will be one nurse to one patient if a patient becomes unstable and requires transfer to a higher level of care.

    - A patient may be what is termed "Fast tracked". This occurs when a patient bypasses phase one recovery and sent directly to phase two recovery. The patient is awake or easily arousable, on room air or at baseline, has minimal pain and is hemodynamically stable.

- Extended care. This is an area where patients require extended observation after discharge from phase 2.

    - Staffing for extended care should be one nurse to three to five patients. These patients are typically awaiting transport home or being held due to waiting to be transported to an inpatient bed.

    - Two staff members should be in the unit at all times. One staff member is a RN who is competent in caring for the patient population.

- Blended Care. This environment involves the care of patients who belong in multiple phases of care. Clinical judgement is required to determine safe staffing levels. Patients in different levels of care may share the same physical space. An effort must be made to ensure privacy and confidentiality of all patients.

Patient Care

Legal forms and Orders

If the patient has a Do Not Resuscitate (DNR) order preoperatively, the surgeon will ask the patient if this continues throughout the perioperative process.

- Living will- the patient has made future healthcare decisions for themselves in the event they become incapacitated and cannot speak for themselves. May be called advance directive.

- Durable power of attorney- The patient has named someone to be their proxy in the event the patient cannot speak for themselves.

- AND- Allow natural death. Comfort measures only.

- POLST- A physician's order regarding life sustaining treatment.

- PSDA- Patient Self Determination Act- The patient is required by law to receive information about advanced directives.

- State Nursing Boards define the Nurses scope of practice within the state.

- Malpractice
    - Failure to provide care that meets the required standard of care.
    - An act of negligence or omission that deviates from the accepted level of care that harms a patient.

- Negligence
    - Duty exists between Parties.
    - Breach of duty.
    - Breach of duty is cause of injury.
    - Injuries or harm occur.
    - Failure to provide care in a way a reasonable person would.

➢ Children are considered emancipated minors when they are married, have a child of their own or are in the military. These patients are no longer reliant on parental control.

- Informed consent- The surgeon explains the following:

    - Diagnosis
    - Procedure
    - Risks
    - Benefits
    - Alternatives

- Evidence – based practice

    - Assists with clinical decision making using a problem-solving approach.
    - Analysis of research
    - Nursing and other clinical expertise
    - Best evidence
    - The goal is to improve patient outcomes.
    - There are three levels of evidence when preparing for recommendations.
        - A- Multiple randomized trials
        - B- Single randomized trials or nonrandomized trials
        - C-Expert opinions, case studies

NPO guidelines:

2 hours clear liquids
4 hours breast milk
6 hours infant formula
6 hours nonhuman milk
6 hours light meal.

- Post-op nausea and vomiting non-medical treatments can include:

    - Aromatherapy with ginger, tarragon, peppermint, or alcohol.

    - Supplemental O2.

    - Deep breathing

Culture of Safety

- A culture of safety involves effective communication. Using checklists and standardized communication tools increases patient safety. An example of standardized communication is the SBAR tool.
  The Joint Commission on Accreditation of Healthcare Organizations (JCAHO) has stated the importance of using standardized communication techniques to improve patient safety. There are many communication tools.

    - I PASS the BATON

      Intro
      Patient
      Assessment
      Situation
      Safety concerns
      Background
      Actions
      Timing
      Ownership
      Next

    - SBAR

      Situation
      Background
      Assessment
      Recommendation

    - Ticket to Ride
      Communication tool commonly used to give information to transporter when the patient is moving to another unit. This information can include information such as if the patient needs oxygen and when the last pain medication was given.

    - Time out
      A "time out" is performed before a procedure is started. All team members stop and listen. The patient, procedure, where the procedure is being performed and other important information is relayed to the team. Every team member is given the opportunity to speak up with any questions or concerns. When the procedure is complete, a debriefing is performed.

Normal vital signs

> Frequency of vital signs is specific to the facility. Vital signs are most commonly collected every five to fifteen minutes in the phase 1. Vital signs in phase 2 range from every 30 to 60 minutes. At a minimum, it is recommended vital signs be taken on arrival and at discharge from phase 2.

- Temperature- 36-38

- B/P
    - Toddler- B/P 95-105 / 55-66
    - Preschooler- B/P 95-110 / 56-70
    - School age child- B/P 97-112 / 57-71
    - Adolescent- B/P 112-128 / 66-80

- HR
    - Age 1-2= 80-130
    - Age 3-4= 80-120
    - Age 5-6= 75-115
    - Age 7-9= 70-110

- Respiratory rate
    - Newborn- 36-60
    - Toddler- 24-40
    - Preschool 22-34
    - School age 18-30

> Capnography: End tidal CO_2- 35-45 measured with capnography

- Can detect early hypoxia to allow correction of hypoventilation, apnea, or airway obstruction.

- Can be used in areas other than the operating room for procedures or peripheral nerve blocks.

- Can increase safety for patients when included with use of pulse oximetry. Oxygen supplementation may correct for pulse oximetry readings but may mask hypoventilation.

> Hemodynamic monitoring- The most common invasive measurements in the PACU are central venous pressure -CVP and arterial blood pressures.

- The CVP measures the pressure in the vena cava and is an estimate of preload and right atrial pressure. The CVP can be used to assess vascular volume and cardiac function. Normal values are 3-8 cmH2O. A CVP can be monitored through a central line. This is attached to a pressure line that needs to be zeroed. Transducer placement is important to obtain correct measurements. Venous blood can be drawn from this pressure line.

- Arterial blood pressures are obtained through an arterial catheter usually placed in the wrist or groin. These are pressure lines that need to be zeroed. Arterial blood gas measurements can be drawn from this pressure line.

- The transducer for CVP and arterial blood pressure measurements should be placed at the mid-anterior-posterior diameter of the chest wall at the fourth intercostal space. An easy way to remember this is it is near where the distal edge of the blood pressure cuff would be on the arm. This area is called the phlebostatic axis which is at the level of the right atrium. The bed should be elevated 60 degrees or less

- Patients may be monitored with a Swan-Ganz catheter which is also known as a right heart catheter or a pulmonary artery catheter. Care must be taken to prevent infections. When checking wedge pressures, be sure not to leave the balloon inflated, this can cause necrosis. The following are some normal values when providing invasive hemodynamic monitoring.

    o Right arterial pressure (RAP) - 2-6 mmHg
    o Right ventricular pressure (RVP)- Systolic-15-25 mmHg, diastolic 0-8
    o Pulmonary artery pressure (PAP)- Systolic15-25 mmHg, Diastolic 8-15
    o Pulmonary artery wedge pressure (PAWP)- 6-12 mmHg
    o Cardiac output (CO)- 4-8 L/min
    o Cardiac index (CI)- 2.5-4 L/min/m2
    o Stroke volume index (SVI) 33-47 ml/m2/beat
    o Systemic vascular resistance (SVR)- 800-1200 dynes

- ICP- Intercranial pressure, can also be monitored in the PACU. The surgeon places a sensor into the patient's skull that is attached to a monitor. Usually there is a device that allows CSF- cerebral spinal fluid- to be drained off if the ICP becomes elevated. The placement of the transducer for ICP measurements is at the tragus of the ear. Normal ICP measures 7 – 15 mm Hg.

- Alarm fatigue is considered a significant safety concern. Several agencies, including the Joint Commission, have indicated alarm fatigue as a potential for patient injury or death. The constant noise due to multiple alarms can cause nurses to change settings without changing back when appropriate, ignore alarms or turn off alarms. The nurse may ignore alarms due to "The boy who cried wolf". Approximately 72 to 99% of alarms have been found to be false in studies.

   Factors related to alarms that have contributed to sentinel events:
   - Deactivation of alarms
   - Lowering of alarm volumes
   - Increased false alarms or unnecessary alarms.
   - Incorrect use of device.

   Recommendations to combat alarm fatigue:
   - Identify important alarms.
   - Develop policies that identify when alarms can be disabled.
   - Use alarms that change back to default settings when the patient is discharged from device.
   - Adjust the alarms to the patient needs.

Normal lab values

- Hemoglobin males- 14-18
- Hemoglobin females- 12-16
- Hematocrit males- 42-52
- Hematocrit females- 37-47
- K- 3.5-5
- NA- 135-145
- Glucose- 70-110
- WBC- 5-10
- Troponin- 0-0.015
- INR- 1.1 or below
- Platelet -150,000 to 450,000
- Calcium- 8.5-10.2
- PH- 7.38-7.11
- PaCo2- 38-42
- Pao2- 75-100
- HCo3- 23-5
- Magnesium- 1.5-2.2 mEq/L
- Albumin- 3.5-5.5 g/dl
- Troponin- I- 0-0.1 ng/ml- peak 10-24 hours, return to normal in 10 to 14 days after cardiac event.

Sedation and Nerve Blocks

- Sedation:
  - Minimal sedation, anxiolysis: Patient responds normally. Coordination may be impaired. Patient able to maintain airway.

  - Moderate sedation, analgesia: Also known as conscious sedation. Patient has a depressed level of consciousness but can respond to verbal commands or light touch. Patient can maintain their own airway.

  - Deep sedation, analgesia: Patient responds purposefully to painful stimulation. The patient may not be able to maintain their own airway.

  - Anesthesia: General anesthesia- the patient loses consciousness, patients are not arousable, usually cannot maintain airway and ventilatory function. Cardiovascular function may be compromised.

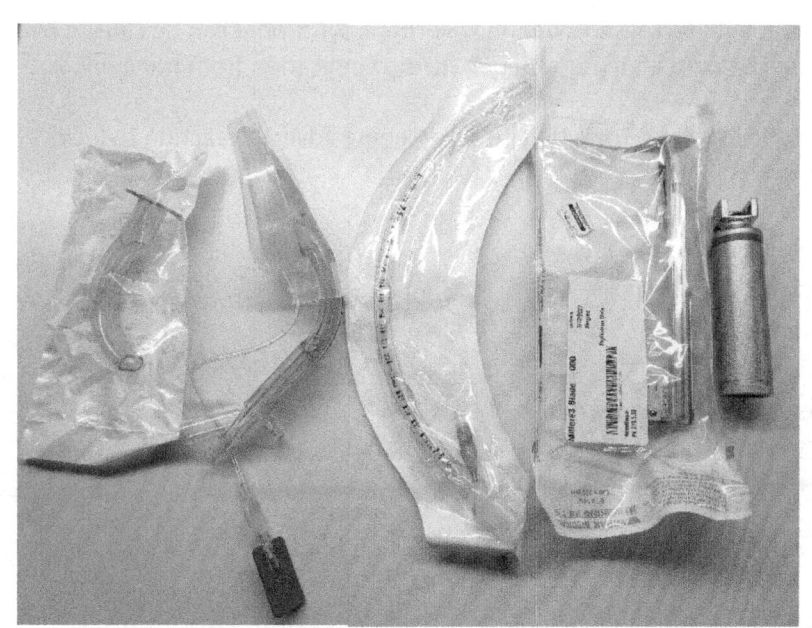

OPA- oropharyngeal airway, LMA- Laryngeal mask airway- do not pass the glottis so is less invasive than the ET but has a higher risk for aspiration, ET- Endotracheal tube, Laryngoscope and blade. Miller blades are straight, Macintosh blades are curved.

- Three phases of general anesthesia- Induction, maintenance, and emergence.

- Oropharyngeal airway- How to measure- Place on cheek, measure distance from corner of mouth to the tragus of the ear.

- Nasopharyngeal airway- How to measure- Nares to the tragus of ear.

- Regional anesthesia: Loss of sensation to specific region of the body. Spinal, epidural, and peripheral nerve blocks are examples.

    - Upper extremity: Brachial plexus blocks for surgery of the shoulder, forearm, or hand. These include: interscalene, supraclavicular, infraclavicular, and axillary.
    - Lower extremity: Femoral, ankle block, and popliteal are examples.

- Local anesthesia: Local infiltration or topical application of anesthetic agent. An anesthesiologist is usually not needed for these minor procedures.

➢ Horner's syndrome- a sign of a medical issue that has caused nerve damage. The nerve from the eye and face to the brain can be damaged and cause drooping eye lid, decreased pupil size, and decreased sweating. Horner's syndrome can be caused by a tumor, stroke, or spinal cord injury or as a negative complication from nerve blocks.

➢ LAST-Local anesthetic Systemic Toxicity- Life threatening adverse reaction to local anesthetics.

- Metallic taste in mouth
- Periorbital numbness
- Tinnitus
- Dysarthria
- Treat with 20% lipid emulsion.
- ACLS

➢ Nerve blocks:

- Retrobulbar- Eye

- Intercostal- nerves that supply the ribs and abdominal wall.

- Bier's block-Tourniquet placed on arm above surgical site. Medication is placed into an IV placed near surgical site.

- Brachial plexus- spinal nerves from C5-T1 vertebrae. Each bundle divides and eventually end in radial, ulnar, and median nerves. Brachial plexus blocks are used for surgeries of the shoulder, forearm, or hand.
    - Interscalene- Shoulder surgeries, upper arm
    - Supraclavicular- Elbow and hand
    - Infraclavicular- Elbow, forearm and hand, but nor shoulder
    - Axillary- forearm wrist or hand

- Lower extremity nerve blocks performed for knee and foot surgeries. Lumbar and sacral nerves divide into sciatic, femoral, popliteal, and tibial nerves.
    - Femoral
    - Ankle

- Abdominal surgeries:
    - Transverse abdominis plane block (TAP).
    - Quadratus lumborum (QL)

To be completed prior to sedation:
- Pre-sedation evaluation by anesthesia provider
- Informed consent
- Nurse relieved of all responsibilities that would prevent that nurse from the ability to constantly monitor sedated patient.
- Sedation scales:
    - POSS: Pasero Opioid Induced Sedation Scale- Evaluates sedation, assesses for unwanted sedation. Research has shown this to be the most reliable scoring system based or reliability and validity and ease of use for nurses.
    - RASS: Richmond Agitation and Sedation Scale- Assessment of sedation in critically ill patients, measures sedation.
    - Aldrete: Determine patients' readiness for discharge from PACU.
    - Ramsey/Modified Ramsey: Assessment of sedation in critically ill patients.
    - Sedation Agitation scale: Assessment of sedation in critically ill patients.

OSA-

Obstructive Sleep Apnea. Airway obstruction during sleep due to reduced muscle tone in the airway.

- Higher incidence in obese patients.
- Increases risk for post-op complications.
- Occurs in 1-5% of general population.

Testing For OSA:

- Sleep study or polysomnography- considered the gold standard for OSA testing. This test can be expensive and requires the patient to spend the night hooked up to machinery in a lab.

- Berlin Questionnaire- The patient answers questions to help determine risk of OSA.

- STOP BANG- Acronym for:

    - Snore
    - Tired
    - Observed- patients family have observed apnea while sleeping.
    - Pressure- Is the patients' blood pressure high?
    - Body mass index- over 35?
    - Age- Over 50?
    - Neck size- 16 inches or larger?
    - Gender- Male?

OSA care considerations:

- Patient may have more frequent desaturations.

- Patient may require extended monitoring.

- Positioning- avoid supine if possible. Sitting or lateral preferred.

- Consider using noninvasive positive pressure ventilation, or CPAP.

    - CPAP- Delivers PEEP, delivers constant pressure.

    - BiPAP- Delivers PEEP, pressure support and timed breaths. Reacts to changes in breathing. Non-invasive equivalent to a ventilator.

- Consider multimodal medications and treatments for pain such as nerve blocks or non-pharmaceutical such as ice.

- If on a PCA, basal is not recommended.

- Facility policy may require patients with OSA to be monitored longer. For example, a patient with OSA may be required to stay in recovery 4 hours post last anesthesia medication before discharge home.

Scoring tools

- FLACC pain scale- used to assess pain in children aged 2 months to 7 years.
    - Face
    - Legs
    - Activity
    - Cry
    - Consolability

- Wong-Baker pain scale- Happy face changing to crying face. Rates on a 0-10 pain scale.

- Braden scale is a tool to help determine pressure sore risks. This is scored by assessing moisture, activity, mobility, nutrition, friction and shear, sensory perception.

- Aldrete score- this tool is most often used in the phase 1 recovery.
    - Activity
        2- Able to move all extremities spontaneously or on command
        1- Able to move 2 extremities spontaneously or on command.
        0- Unable to move any extremities.

    - Respiration
        2- Able to deep breath and cough
        1- Dyspnea, limited breathing
        0- Apneic

    - Circulation
        2- B/P within 20 mmHg of pre-op level

1- B/P within 20-50 mmHg of pre-op level

0- B/P more than 50 mmHg change from pre-op level

- Consciousness

    2- Fully awake

    1- Awake on calling.

    0- Not responsive

- Skin color

    2- Normal

    1- Pale, dusky, jaundiced.

    0- Cyanotic

Modified Aldrete score replaces skin color with oxygen saturation.

- Oxygen saturation

    2- SpO2 greater than 92% on room air

    1- SpO2 greater than 90% with supplemental oxygen

    0- SpO2 less than 90% even with supplemental O2

➢ Glasgow coma scale

- Eye opening response

    4- Spontaneous

    3- To verbal stimuli

    2- To pain

    1- No response

- Verbal response

    5- Oriented

    4- Confused but able to answer questions

    3- Inappropriate words

    2- Speech incomprehensible

    1- No response

- Motor response

    6- Obeys commands for movement

    5- Responds purposefully to painful stimuli

    4- Withdraws from pain

    3- Flexion in response to painful stimuli

    2- Decerebrate posturing to pain.

    1- No response to pain

> ASA- American Society of Anesthesiology uses a classification system to score patients based on physiological conditions that are not related to the surgery. This may also be seen as a PS- physical status classification.

    ASA 1 - is a healthy non-smoking, normal BMI patient.

    ASA 2 - is a patient with mild diseases but well controlled/ may be a Current smoker. BMI 30 to 40.

    ASA 3 - is a patient with severe systemic disease such as COPD or poorly controlled Diabetes.

    ASA 4 - is a patient with a disease that is a constant threat to life. This could patient with recent CVA or MI.

    ASA 5 - is a patient not expected to survive without the planned Surgery

    ASA 6 - is a brain-dead patient waiting for organ harvest.

Emergency Situations

Malignant Hyperthermia-

Caused by an autosomal dominate trait, causes calcium to be released from muscles. Triggered by Succinylcholine and isoflurane, halothane, sevoflurane, desflurane. Nitrous oxide, propofol and midazolam are safe. Family history is taken pre-op to see if there are any unusual surgical deaths or if malignant hyperthermia is known. A muscle biopsy is the procedure for diagnosis preoperatively.

- S/S:
    - Tachycardia
    - Co2 absorber becomes blue and heated.
    - Tachypnea
    - Increased end tidal CO2
    - Muscle rigidity
    - Mottling of skin
    - Hyperthermia
    - Increased potassium
    - Myoglobinuria
    - Hypertension
    - Increased minute ventilation

- Treatment:
    - Dantrolene (Ryanodex)- 2.5 mg/kg. Repeat until 10mg/kg. Only dilute with preservative free sterile water. Dantrolene is a hydantoin skeletal muscle relaxant that also effects the vascular and heart muscle.
    - Ice packs
    - Cold IV solution.
    - Treating symptoms- electrolyte imbalances, cardiac dysrhythmias.

- Medications that do not cause malignant hyperthermia:
    - Nitrous oxide
    - Opioids
    - Barbiturates

- Droperidol
- Propofol
- Benzodiazepines
- Ketamine
- Etomidate

- Medications that may activate malignant hyperthermia:
    - Halothane
    - Enflurane
    - Isoflurane
    - Sevoflurane
    - Desflurane

Blood transfusion reaction

- Fever
- Rash
- Dyspnea
- Hypotension
- Bronchospasm
- Anxiety
- Increased interop bleeding
- Weak pulse
- Vasomotor instability
- Decreased urine output.

Special Patient Considerations

Pregnancy

- Increased cardiac output- 30 to 50%
- Increased HR
- Increased breathing and increased tidal volume.
- Increased blood glucose
- Decreased gastric motility- can increase risk for aspiration.
- Pregnancy risks for surgery:

    - Preeclampsia- Magnesium given IV to prevent seizures. Magnesium may cause an increased risk of respiratory depression.

    - Post -op cesarean delivery the uterus should be firm and midline. Oxytocin increases uterine contractions and can stop bleeding.

    - Post-delivery the lochia should be dark- rubra- or bright red, with clots. The absence of clots could indicate disseminated intravascular coagulation, DIC.

    - Post-partum hemorrhage is considered more than 500 ML of blood. The first signs of hemorrhagic shock in these patients may be mild tachycardia.

The Elderly

- Normal changes include:
    - Increase in body fat.
    - Arteriosclerotic changes, valvular compliance, coronary artery flow
    - Delayed drug metabolism. Can cause delayed anesthesia awakening.
    - Decrease in cardiac output.
    - Decreased renal perfusion.
    - Increased risk of clotting disorders such as DVT and stroke.

Infants and children

- Increased surface area decreased mass; Lack of subcutaneous fat can contribute to hypothermia.
- Decreased functional residual capacity.
- Decreased o2 reserves.
- Greater o2 consumption.
- Greater metabolic rate.
- Infants are nose breathers, large tongue, narrow nasal passages, short neck.

Medications

- ➤ Pain medications

  - Acetaminophen- non -opioid, adults should not take more than 4000 mg per 24 hours. Can be toxic to liver.
  - Celebrex- Can be given pre-op to help prevent post op pain.
  - Hydromorphone (Dilaudid)- analgesic opioid agonist.
  - Fentanyl- Analgesic opioid agonists
  - Meperidine (Demerol)- Can be used for patients shivering post op.
  - Morphine
  - Norco- Acetaminophen plus hydrocodone. Opioid for moderate to moderate sever pain.
  - NSAID
  - Oxycodone
  - Tramadol- Ultram- Analgesic opioid agonists, treats moderate to severe pain.
  - Aspirin- Some patients may take this for pain control. Aspirin inhibits prostaglandin synthesis. Platelets are disabled. Should be stopped before surgery. Platelets can be infused to revers effects.
  - Ketorolac (Toradol)- NSAID analgesic.

- ➤ Anesthesia gasses

  - Desflurane- Fluorinated methyl ether, general anesthetic
  - Halothane- General anesthetic
  - Isoflurane (Forane)-General anesthetic
  - Nitrous oxide- Anesthetic gas with pain reliving properties.
  - Sevoflurane- Fluorinated isopropyl ether, general anesthetic

- ➤ Neuromuscular blocking agents, paralytics

  - Nimbex (Cisatracurium)- Non-depolarizing neuromuscular blocker.
  - Pavulon (Pancuronium)- can increase heart rate, increase cardiac output, and increase mean arterial pressure (MAP).
  - Rocuronium- non-depolarizing neuromuscular blocker.
  - Anectine (Succinylcholine)- depolarizing agent.
  - Norcuron (Vecuronium)- Has minimal hemodynamic effects.

- Local Anesthetics

  - Bupivacaine
  - Epinephrine- alpha/ beta agonist. Added to other local medications to increase duration of the anesthetic effect.
  - Lidocaine
  - Tetracaine
  - Cocaine- Topical anesthetic, vasoconstrictor.

- Treatment for hypertension

  - Nitroprusside (Nipride)
  - Hydralazine (Apresoline)
  - Vasotec
  - Nifedipine
  - Labetalol
  - Amidate (Etomidate)- decreases blood pressure.

- Antiemetics

  - Droperidol- Antiemetic with sedative and anti- anxiety effects.
  - Metoclopramide
  - Ondansetron
  - Promethazine
  - Scopolamine- Patch placed behind ear to help prevent surgical nausea and vomiting. Can also be given to reduce saliva. Anticholinergic drug. Also known as Devils breath. That won't be on the test, its just cool.
  - Dexamethasone

- Reversal agents

  - Flumazenil- Reverses effects of benzodiazepines.
  - Narcan- Opioid antagonist.
  - Sugammadex- Neuromuscular reversal drug. Female patients of childbearing age should be cautioned to use a back-up birth control method if on birth control pills.
  - Protamine- reverse effects of heparin. Derived from fish. Can cause Hypotension and pulmonary hypertension.
  - Vitamin K- reverse effects of Coumadin- Warfarin

- Anticoagulants
    - Coumadin- warfarin
    - Heparin
    - Clopidogrel- often used for patients with coronary stents

- Antibiotics
    - Cefazolin
    - Ceftriaxone
    - Ciprofloxacin
    - Gentamycin
    - Imipenem
    - Metronidazole
    - Vancomycin

- Diuretics
    - Bumetanide (Bumex)- Loop diuretic
    - Ethacrynic acid (Edecrin)- Loop diuretic
    - Furosemide (Lasix)- Loop diuretic
    - Mannitol (Osmitrol)- Osmotic diuretic
    - Torsemide (Demadex)- Loop diuretic

- Herbs
    - St. Johns wart- may prolong anesthesia.
    - Garlic, ginkgo, ginger- May cause post-op bleeding.
    - Ginseng- Can increase blood pressure and heart rate.
    - Valerian- Can increase effects of anesthesia and prolong patient recovery and "Wake up" from surgery.

- Anti-hypertensives
    - Hydralazine- Treats hypertension, direct acting vasodilator
    - Sodium nitroprusside- Used to treat hypertension, vasodilator
    - Magnesium- Can be given via IV for hypertension, common in post-delivery in women.

- Miscellaneous
  - Dantrolene- Treatment for malignant hyperthermia
  - Glycopyrrolate- Reduces secretions. Anticholinergic. Used to control heart rate. Non-surgical use includes control of peptic ulcers. Anticholinergic drugs can cause tachycardia, dry mouth.
  - Hetastarch (Hespan)- Plasma expander.
  - Ketalar (Ketamine)- Dissociative anesthetic. Can increase heart rate and blood pressure. Can cause hallucinations.
  - Metoprolol- Beta blocker
  - Midazolam (Versed)- Benzodiazepine, anticonvulsant, sedative-hypnotic.
  - Nitroglycerine- Used to prevent chest pain, can lower blood pressure.
  - Oxytocin (Pitocin)- Help the uterus contract after delivery.
  - Phenylephrine (Neo-Synephrine)- Alpha adrenergic. Causes vasoconstriction, decreased heart rate, increased blood pressure.
  - Precedex (Dexmedetomidine)- sedative, hypnotic. Relaxes smooth muscle.
  - Diprivan (Propofol)- Short acting, causes loss of consciousness and lack of memory. Can be given In an IV drip for patient on ventilators in the ICU.
  - RhoGAM- Derived from human plasma. Helps prevent Rh immunization also called Rh incompatibility. Given to people who are Rh negative but receives blood products that are Rh positive or to women who are Rh neg and may be pregnant with a fetus who is Rh positive.
  - Rifampin- Can be given to TB patients. Can turn urine, tears, and other secretions orange.
  - SSRI- Selective serotonin reuptake inhibitors. These medications may slow hepatic clearance of anesthetic drugs.
  - Tranexamic acid- Helps decrease blood loss. Inhibits fibrinolysis.

CAPA Example Questions

1) You are working in the pre-operative unit preparing a patient for a bowel resection. The anesthesiologist tells you she will be in soon to perform an Allan's test. You know this test is for:

   A) To determine the patency of the ulnar artery.

   B) To determine the patency of the radial artery.

   C) To assess the total lung volume.

   D) To determine exercise tolerance.

2) A patient presents to the emergency room with abdominal pain. The surgeon determines the patient requires a bowel resection. You are asked to pre-op the patient. You are old by the emergency room nurse that the patient's primary language is not English. What is your response?

   A) You will use the patient's family as interpreters.

   B) You will simply gesture and point a lot.

   C) Contact an interpreter that is contracted with the facility.

   D) Find the nurse you know who speaks a little of the patient's language.

3) Your patient is in the pre-op holding area ready for surgery. The patient asks the pre-op nurse about specific complications that could occur related to the procedure. What should the nurse do?

   A) Answer he patient.

   B) Ask the charge nurse to talk to the patient.

   C) Tell the patient they can ask the surgeon after he procedure.

   D) Call the surgeon to come talk to the patient.

4) You are taking a history on a patient pre-operatively. You are asking about medications when the patient tells you he took his metformin right before leaving home to the hospital. What should your response be?

   A) Metformin is allowed the morning of surgery.

   B) Notify the Surgeon.

   C) The surgery will be delayed until later in the day.

   D) Plan to give glucagon pre-op.

5) Your pre-op patient is very anxious about post-op pain. You know all the following education may help your patient except:

   A) Teach target relaxation techniques.

   B) Tell your patient there will be no pain.

   C) Tell the patient approximately how long the pain will last.

   D) Involve the patient in pain management techniques.

6) Your patient had lumbar spinal fusion. Which of the following will you include in your post-op teaching?

   A) Bend at the knees not at the waist.

   B) Use a soft cushion when sitting.

   C) Start back exercises the day after surgery.

   D) Sleep on your stomach.

7) Your patient is complaining of an earache after a tonsillectomy. What is your response?

   A) This is abnormal, notify the surgeon.

   B) This indicates an infection.

   C) This is normal. Give Ibuprofen for pain.

   D) This is normal. Give Tylenol for pain.

8) Which of the following would you not include in your post op teaching for a patient having a septoplasty?

   A) Do not blow your nose for 2 weeks.

   B) Sleep with head elevated.

   C) Take Ibuprofen, aspirin or Tylenol for pain.

   D) Headaches and congestion are normal.

9) Which of the following would you include in post-op instructions for sclerotherapy?

   A) Keep legs elevated as much as possible day of procedure.

   B) Take ibuprofen for discomfort.

   C) Remove bandages after 1 week.

   D) Walk as much as possible the day after surgery.

10) You are asked to assist with a pain block in the operating room. The patient is scheduled to receive abdominal surgery for colon cancer. What type of pain block is the patient probably going to receive?

   A) Interscalene

   B) TAP block

   C) Sphenopalatine

   D) Retrobulbar

11) Which of the following would you not include in discharge instructions for a patient going home with a scopolamine patch?

   A) Wash hands after handling the patch.

   B) Do not use the patch if you have narrow angle glaucoma.

   C) The patch can be left on for 2 weeks.

   D) The patch can cause dry mouth.

12) Which of the following pharmacological treatments for post op nausea and vomiting is a corticosteroid?

   A) Zofran

   B) Anzemet

   C) Kytril

   D) Decadron

13) Which of the following is a risk factor for post op nausea and vomiting?

   A) Male gender

   B) Patients who smoke.

   C) Short surgical times.

   D) Female

14) Potential side effects of dexamethasone could be all the following except:

   A) Decreased blood sugar

   B) Increased blood sugar

   C) Fluid retention

   D) Delayed wound healing

15) Heat loss to surrounding air is called:

   A) Evaporation

   B) Convection

   C) Radiation

   D) Conduction

16) What is not true of an arteriovenous shunt?

   A) Can be used immediately.

   B) Cannot be used immediately.

   C) Generally placed in forearm, wrist or upper arm.

   D) A thrill over the site should be palpable.

17) ESWL- Extracorporeal shock wave lithotripsy is for what purpose?

   A) Provide back pain relief.

   B) Permanent birth control.

   C) Plastic surgery procedure to remove unwanted adipose tissue.

   D) Procedure to break up renal calculi.

18) Post op instructions for a patient who has had an ESWL would include all the following except:

   A) Brusing on flank is normal.

   B) Drink plenty of fluids post op.

   C) Pink urine is not normal, call the doctor.

   D) Stain urine post op and take any fragments of stone to doctor appointment.

19) An orchiectomy is:

   A) Removal of an ovary

   B) Removal of eye

   C) Removal of testicle

   D) Entering an organ with a trocar and endoscope

20) The Raz sling, Stamey and Burch procedures correct what condition?

   A) Urinary stress incontinence

   B) Infertility

   C) Undescended testicles

   D) Rotator cuff repair

21) Which of the following would be included in post op instructions after a nasal surgery?

   A) Lay flat when sleeping

   B) Encourage mouth breathing

   C) Blow nose as needed

   D) Drink with a straw

22) Patient education for post op care after tonsillectomy would not include:

   A) Pain may increase between days 4 to 8 post op.

   B) Eat a soft bland diet.

   C) Minimize talking.

   D) Stay NPO for 24 hours post op.

23) Your patient states he had a large breakfast with eggs and bacon at 0600 this morning. What is the earliest time he can have his nonemergent surgery?

   A) 1100

   B) 1200

   C) 1400

   D) 1800

24) A defect involving herniation of small intestine into the vaginal wall is called:

   A) Urethrocele

   B) Enterocele

   C) Rectocele

   D) Cystocele

25) Which of the following is a set of questions used to assess for obstructive sleep apnea- OSA?

   A) STOP-BANG

   B) Wong Baker

   C) FLACC

   D) Aldrete

CAPA Example Questions Answers and Rationales

1) A
   The Allen's test is used to determine the patency of the ulnar artery. This is done prior to the placement of an arterial line to make sure the hand will still be perfused if the radial artery is damaged.

2) C
   For patients who do not speak English, a official contracted interpreter is preferred.

3) D
   Questions about the procedure need to be answered before the procedure by the surgeon. This is a part of informed consent.

4) B
   Metformin is usually held prior to surgery due to metformin preventing the liver in metabolizing lactic acid efficiently. For large surgeries such as when a large amount of tissue damage is expected or when tourniquets or clamps are used, metformin can be held up to 36 hours before surgery. Metformin induced lactic acidosis can be fatal.

5) B
   The patient may be less distressed by post-op pain if it is expected.

6) A
   After spinal fusion surgery it is recommended to bend at the knees not at the waist. Soft cushions do not offer enough support when sitting. Start exercises 3 to 4 weeks post op. Do not lay on stomach or twist spine when sleeping. Place pillow between legs to help prevent moving to stomach or turning when sleeping.

7) D
   An earache is normal after a tonsillectomy. Do not give Ibuprofen, this medication can cause increased bleeding.

8) C
   Do not take Ibuprofen or aspirin. These medications could cause increased bleeding.

9) A
   For pain control, take Tylenol. Aspirin and ibuprofen may cause increased bleeding. Remove bandages after 48 hours. Resume normal activity after 48 hours, not 24.

10) B

A TAP block- transversus abdominus plane block, is for abdominal surgeries. A sphenopalatine block is for the nose and palate. An interscalene block is for the upper extremity such as for a rotator cuff repair.

11) C

The patch can be left on for up to 72 hours.

12) D

Decadron is a corticosteroid.

13) D

Risk factors for post op nausea and vomiting include female gender, non-smokers, long surgical times and patients who suffer from motion sickness.

14) A

Dexamethasone can increase blood sugar.

15) B

Evaporation is caused by sweating, exhaling, insatiable fluid loss. Conduction is loss to other objects such as the OR table or cold blankets. Radiation is heat loss to another object with no physical contact.

16) A

AV shunts cannot be used immediate. The shunt needs to heal.

17) D

ESWL is used to break up renal calculi.

18) C

Pink urine is normal after ESWL.

19) C

Orchiectomy is removal of a testicle.

20) A

The Raz sling, Stamey and Burch procedure correct urinary incontinence.

21) B

The patient should not use a straw after nasal surgery, blow nose or lay flat.

22) D

The patient may eat soft bland foods the day of surgery. The patient may be given ice chips as soon as they can tolerate po.

23) C

Patients typically need to be NPO for 8 hours after a large meal before surgery.

24) B

A urethrocele is a protrusion of urethral tissues into the vagina. A rectocele is the protrusion of the rectum into the vagina. A cystocele is the bladder causing the vagina wall to bulge down.

25) A

The Wong Baker and FLACC scales are used for pain assessment. The Aldrete scale is used to determine readiness to discharge from PACU.

CPAN Example Questions

1) The phase 1 nurse extubates a patient post bowel resection. The nurse notes strider when auscultation breath sounds. What action should the nurse take?

   A) Raise the patient's head

   B) Notify the anesthesia provider

   C) Suction the patient

   D) Place o2 per nasal canula.

2) All of the following can be typically seen with thyroid storm except:

   A) Bradycardia

   B) Fever

   C) Tachycardia

   D) Hypertension

3) Which of the following lab values would be seen on a hypoxic patient?

   A) PaO2 100 mm Hg

   B) PaO2 90 mmHg

   C) PaO2 80 mmHg

   D) PaO2 70 mm Hg

4) Cheyne-Stoke breathing after neurosurgery can be a sign of:

    A) Decreased intracranial pressure

    B) Increased intracranial pressure

    C) A normal sign

    D) A sign of pain.

5) The phase 1 PACU nurse receives a patient from the operating room with a central venous pressure monitor in place. The nurse is told to watch for signs of cardiac tamponade. Which of the following could indicate a cardiac tamponade?

    A) Central venous pressure is not affected by cardiac tamponade.

    B) The central venous pressure will decrease.

    C) The central venous pressure will increase.

    D) The only way to determine a cardiac tamponade is if the central venous catheter is also connected to a pulmonary artery catheter.

6) Your patient in phase 1 recovery is showing signs of myocardial ischemia. The patient is complaining of chest pain and has ST changes on EKG. The anesthesiologist gives nitroglycerine. The patient then develops a reflex tachycardia. What medication do you expect to be given next?

    A) Hydralazine

    B) Propofol

    C) Epinephrine

    D) Metoprolol

7) Which of the following medications would you not expect to give to a hypertensive patient?

   A) Ephedrine

   B) Clonidine

   C) Nitroprusside

   D) Labetalol

8) Which of the following is a normal pH on an arterial blood gas reading?

   A) 7.25 - 7.35

   B) 7.35 - 7.45

   C) 7.45 - 7.55

   D) 7.55 - 7.65

9) You just received a patient with an oral airway in place from the operating room. The patient is not arousable but hemodynamically stable. The charge nurse asks if the only other nurse working in the PACU to go to another department to give a break. What is your response?

   A) This is fine because the nurse will be available via phone if you need help.

   B) This is fine because the operating room is just past the double doors. They will be able to hear you if you yell really loud.

   C) You are adequately staffed because you have the junior volunteer at the desk.

   D) You cannot let the other nurse go unless another nurse takes her place to stay with you.

10) What is the most commonly accepted spinal level assessed in a patient to allow discharge from the phase 1 recovery?

   A) T 7

   B) T 8

   C) T 10

   D) C 8

11) Your post op patient is considered hypotensive when their blood pressure falls below what percent of their pre op value?

   A) 5%

   B) 10%

   C) 15%

   D) 20%

12) All the following are medications used to treat hypotension except:

   A) Hydralazine

   B) Epinephrine

   C) Dopamine

   D) Phenylephrine

13) Your patient has a central venous pressure (CVP) monitor in place. The reading is 12 cm H2O. What may this indicate?

   A) Hypovolemia

   B) Hypervolemia

   C) Distributive shock

   D) Hemmorrhage

14) Who is at risk for HELLP syndrome?

    A) Elderly men

    B) Pregnant women

    C) Patients with brain cancer

    D) Children with fractures

15) After assisting with a central line placement in the PACU on an unstable patient, an air embolism is expected. Which of the following would be a correct action?

    A) Turn the patient to right side.

    B) Lay the patient flat

    C) Turn the patient to the left side

    D) Sit the patient upright.

16) Your patient had extensive blood loss during surgery. The patient was given several boluses of lactated ringers, normal saline and blood products. When they come to the PACU, the vital signs are stable. The patient currently is having a unit of blood infusing with normal saline wide open. Which of the following demonstrate a possible fluid overload?

    A) CVP reading of 5 cm H2O

    B) HR decreases from 100 BPM to 90 BPM, Blood pressure 140/85 mmHg

    C) Urine output during surgery 20 ML/HR, has increased to 50 ML/HR

    D) The patient on admit to the PACU had clear breath sounds, now the nurse auscultates crackles.

17) Kussmaul's respiration can be caused by which of the following conditions?

    A) Diabetic ketoacidosis

    B) Cerebral vascular accident- stroke

    C) Injury of the medulla

    D) Cardiac arrest

18) Which of the following is a potential complication caused by hypothermia?

    A) Increased drug metabolism

    B) Promoted bleeding

    C) Decrease blood viscosity

    D) Increased cough reflex

19) At what anatomical level should the transducer be placed for monitoring intercranial pressure- ICP?

    A) Top of frontal lobe

    B) Mid carotid

    C) Center of chin

    D) Tragus of ear

20) A patient presents with a skull fracture sent from the emergency department for emergency surgery. You notice the patient has bruising around the eyes like a racoon. What type of skull fracture presents with this sign?

    A) Linear

    B) Depressed

    C) Basilar

    D) Ovid

21) Drainage of cerebral spinal fluid- CSF, should take place when the ventricular monitor device indicated the intercranial pressure- ICP, is a t what level?

   A) 20 mmHg

   B) 30 m Hg

   C) 40 mm Hg

   D) 50 mm Hg

22) Beck's triad are signs of a cardiac tamponade and include all the following except:

   A) Decreased arterial blood pressure

   B) Increased arterial pressure

   C) Distended jugular veins

   D) Muffled heart sounds

23) Tension pneumothorax can cause what type of shock?

   A) Obstructive

   B) Distributive

   C) Cardiogenic

   D) Neurogenic

24) Virchow's triad which is a group of risk factors for DVT- deep vein thrombosis. This includes all the following except:

   A) Venous stasis

   B) Hypercoagulability

   C) Infection

   D) Friable blood vessel walls

25) Meperidine is contraindicated in patients with what conditions?

   A) Elderly patients

   B) Patients with infections

   C) Patients who have had abdominal surgery

   D) Patients who are on MAOI's

CPAN Example Questions Answers and Rationales

1) B
   The anesthesia provider should be notified when stridor is present. Stridor may indicate laryngeal edema with may necessitate reintubation.

2) A
   Tachycardia, fever and hypertension are commonly seen with thyroid storm.

3) D
   A normal PaO2 is 75 to 100 mm Hg

4) B
   Cheyne-Stoke breathing after neurosurgery can be a sign of increased intracranial pressure. The surgeon should be notified.

5) C
   An indication of a cardiac tamponade is an increase in the central venous pressure.

6) D
   Metoprolol would be most commonly given in the above situation. Hydralazine may also cause reflex tachycardia and ischemia.

7) A
   Ephedrine may increase blood pressure, not decrease it.

8) B
   7.35 – 7.45 is a normal pH on a blood gas result.

9) D
   Per ASPAN standards, two nurses must be in the department with a phase 1 patient.

10) C
    T 10 is considered a safe spinal level to allow the patient to move to a lower level of care.

11) D
    20% drop from pre op blood pressure is considered hypotensive.

12) A
    Hydralazine is used to treat hypertension.

13) B
An elevated CVP reading can indicate hypervolemia, heart failure due to decreased heart contractility, pulmonary artery stenosis, and some dysrhythmias.

14) B
Hemolysis, elevated liver enzymes and low platelets are associated with HELLP syndrome. HELLP syndrome occurs in pregnant women when pre-eclampsia is progressing to eclampsia.

15) C
Turning the patient to their left side may lessen the amount of air entering the pulmonary artery. This is called the Durrants maneuver.

16) D
Crackles in the lungs followed by wheezing can indicate fluid overload.

17) A
Kussmaul's respiration is rapid deep breathing at a constant pace. This is caused by metabolic acidosis. Stroke can cause Cheyne-Soke breathing. Injury to the medulla can cause Biot's breathing which is similar to Cheyne-Stokes. Breathing pattern of cardiac arrest is probably apnea.

18) B
Hypothermia can promote bleeding, decrease drug metabolism, increase blood viscosity and decrease the couch reflex.

19) D
The tragus of the ear is the most common anatomical location to level the transducer for the ICP monitor.

20) C
A basilar skull fracture is commonly seen with "racoon eyes". For linear skull fractures, there is usually no treatment to the being a mild condition. Depressed skull fractures are commonly open with infection being a concern. There is no Ovid fractures.

21) A
20 mm Hg is the level at which drainage of CSF is needed.

22) B
Decreased arterial blood pressure, distended jugular veins and muffled heart sounds are signs of cardiac tamponade.

23) A
Tension pneumothorax can cause obstructive shock. Disruptive shock is a group of shock types- neurogenic, septic and anaphylactic.

24) C
Infection is not part of Virchow's triad.

25) D
Patients on MAOI's and patients who have seizure disorders should not take meperidine. Elderly patients can have meperidine, but it is recommended the dose be lower.

CPAN/CAPA Example Questions

1) What is an example of visceral pain?

    A) Pain from injured nerves.

    B) Sharp pain, muscle, skin, joint pain.

    C) Inflammation irritating pain receptors that lasts for longer than 6 months.

    D) Deep, not localized, from intraabdominal organs.

2) What class of drugs does Flumazenil reverse?

    A) Benzodiazepines

    B) Anesthesia gasses

    C) Opioids

    D) Anticoagulant

3) You are getting report from a nurse who is going on break on a patient who is recovering from surgery who had a spinal anesthesia. The nurse tells you the patient's spinal level is at T 10. You know this correlate to what area of the body?

    A) Nipple

    B) Umbilicus

    C) Hip

    D) Groin

4) Your patient is scheduled for a cholecystectomy. You are asked to help with a nerve block. You know the most common type of block for a cholecystectomy is:

   A) Thoracic paravertebral

   B) Axillary

   C) Supraclavicular

   D) Intercostal

5) What is the action of neuromuscular blocking drugs?

   A) Pain control

   B) Blood pressure regulation

   C) Paralyze skeletal muscle

   D) Heart rate control

6) Which of the following medications would be given to a woman post-delivery to contract her uterus?

   A) Oxytocin

   B) Oxybutynin

   C) Oxycontin

   D) Oxycodone

7) Which of the following situations would you expect to give a belladonna and opium – B & O- suppository?

   A) Constipation

   B) Bladder spasm

   C) To contract the uterus

   D) Prior to hemorrhoid surgery

8) Which of the following is an opioid antagonist?

   A) Norco

   B) Nifedipine

   C) Romazicon

   D) Narcan

9) Which of the following is a calcium channel blocker?

   A) Digoxin

   B) Amiodarone

   C) Metoprolol

   D) Verapamil

10) Which of the following is not a reason to warm blood before transfusion?

    A) Cold blood can clump

    B) Cold blood can cause hypothermia

    C) Cold blood can cause arrhythmias and cause cardiac output to increase

    D) Transfusing cold blood can be painful to the patient

11) What is the purpose for a Whipple procedure?

    A) To resect a carcinoma from the head of the pancreas

    B) To repair a damaged rotator cuff

    C) Emergency surgery on an infant with congenital conditions

    D) To resect a tumor in the frontal lobe of the brain

12) You are asked to go into the operating room to help move a patient from the operating room bed to a stretcher. How many people are needed to move this patient that weighs 100 KG?

    A) Anesthesia provider at head, one person on each side.

    B) Anesthesia at head, one person at each side, one person to hold feet.

    C) Anesthesia at head, one to pull patient to stretcher, one person at feet.

    D) Anesthesia at head, 2 people on each side.

13) Which of the following is responsible for defining and establishing the scope of PeriAnesthesia nursing?

    A) ASPAN

    B) ANA

    C) NLN

    D) SCIP

14) You hear in report that your patient received salvaged autologous blood. You know this to mean:

    A) The patient received blood from a donor that was not cross matched.

    B) The patient received blood from a close relative.

    C) The patient received blood that had a different RH type

    D) The patient's own blood was saved during surgery and reinfused into the patient.

15) You are called in the PACU for a "code blue". When you arrive, you see the patient receiving chest compressions and is intubated. The compressions are stopped for a pulse check. The EKG shows normal sinus rhythm. The nurse and anesthesiologist both check for a pulse and cannot palpate one. What is a likely scenario?

   A) The patient's heart rhythm is probably actually A fib.

   B) A new staff member is needed to find the pulse.

   C) The patient needs to be defibrillated.

   D) The patient is in PEA

16) You are helping with a patient who is in cardiac arrest. The team stops compressions for a pulse check. The anesthesiologist who is team lead for the code decides the patient is in torsade's de points. What medication do you expect to give?

   A) Magnesium

   B) Potassium

   C) Calcium

   D) Sodium bicarbonate

17) Your patient underwent a TURP. The surgeon reminds you to watch for TURP syndrome. You know TURP syndrome includes:

   A) Pian

   B) Bleeding

   C) Hyponatremia

   D) Hypernatremia

18) Signs and symptoms of a hemolytic transfusion reaction are all the following except:

   A) Hypertension, bradycardia

   B) Sudden fever

   C) Chest pain

   D) Hematuria

19) What MAP- mean arterial pressure- measurement is required to maintain adequate tissue perfusion?

   A) 35 mmHg

   B) 45 mmHg

   C) 55 mmHg

   D) 65 mmHg

20) A fasciotomy is done for what condition?

   A) Heart failure

   B) Compartment syndrome

   C) Foot fractures

   D) Pneumothorax

21) Which procedure would be performed for a patient needing a stent placed to relieve bile duct obstruction caused by stones?

   A) ERCP

   B) TIPS

   C) PEG

   D) ICP

22) A patient is brought to the PACU intubated with medications infusing to maintain blood pressure control and sedation. There are two other patients in the PACU. One is waiting for transport to the medical floor, the other is stable with complaints of pain and nausea. What is the appropriate staffing level at this time?

    A) One RN, one assistive staff such as a nurse's aide.

    B) One RN with another RN nearby in the ambulatory care unit.

    C) Two RN's proficient in the care of PACU phase 1 patients

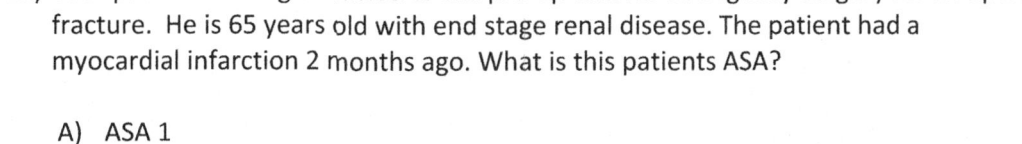

    D) One RN, one student nurse in training.

23) Your patient is being admitted to the pre-op unit for emergency surgery for an open fracture. He is 65 years old with end stage renal disease. The patient had a myocardial infarction 2 months ago. What is this patients ASA?

    A) ASA 1

    B) ASA 2

    C) ASA 3

    D) ASA 4

24) There are five principles that govern the ethics of nursing. Beneficence, autonomy, justice, fidelity and veracity. What is the definition of veracity?

    A) Being kind to all patients

    B) Providing the ability for patients to make their own decisions

    C) Being trustworthy and keeping promises

    D) Fair treatment to all patients

25) You are informed that your patient may have experienced a corneal abrasion during surgery. What will be a part of your discharge teaching?

   A) The cornea will heal on its own in 24 to 72 hours.

   B) Eye surgery will be required to repair the cornea.

   C) Eye drops will be needed for 2 weeks.

   D) The patient may lose their eyesight.

26) The dermatome landmark for T 6-7 is located where?

   A) Knee

   B) Middle finger

   C) Umbilicus

   D) Xiphoid

27) The nurse can prevent ICP from increasing by all the following except:

   A) Maintaining semi- Fowlers position

   B) Lay patient flat

   C) Hyperventilate patient

   D) Pain management

28) What is the difference between CPAP and BiPap?

   A) CPAP delivers PEEP, BiPap does not. CPAP provides constant high pressure, BiPap provides pressure on inspiration, low pressure on expiration.

   B) Both deliver PEEP. CPAP provides constant high pressure, BiPap provides high pressure on inspiration and low pressure on inspiration.

   C) Both deliver PEEP. CPAP provides high pressure only on inspiration and low pressure on expiration, BiPap provides constant pressure.

   D) BiPap delivers PEEP, CPAP does not. CPAP provides constant high pressure, BiPap only provides pressure on inspiration with low pressure on expiration.

29) Which of the following is not part of Cushing's triad?

   A) Tachycardia

   B) Bradycardia

   C) Hypertension

   D) Bradypnea

30) According to ASPAN standards, which of the following is not required in a PACU?

   A) Resuscitation equipment

   B) Equipment to administer blood and IV medications

   C) Compute charting

   D) Appropriate physiological monitoring equipment

31) You are told in report your patient has pseudocholinesterase deficiency. You know this condition involves what?

   A) When the patient has increased sensitivity to propofol.

   B) When the patient has an allergic reaction to propofol.

   C) When the patient has an overdose of nitrous oxide.

   D) When the patient has increased sensitivity to succinylcholine.

32) Your patient received one unit of packed red blood cells- PRBC's. You are expecting the patient's hemoglobin and hematocrit to raise by how much?

   A) Hemoglobin 1 g/dL and Hematocrit 8%

   B) Hemoglobin 1 g/dL and Hematocrit 3%

   C) Hemoglobin 3 g/dL and Hematocrit 8%

   D) Hemoglobin 3 g/dL and Hematocrit 3%

33) Your patient is wheezing and developing inspiratory stridor. You note bradycardia with tracheal deviation. The patient is having trouble moving air. What may be happening?

   A) Laryngospasm

   B) Bronchospasm

   C) Croup

   D) PE

34) Your patient has finished surgery and comes to the PACU arousable and able to maintain their own airway. You are told the patient received Iv propofol and maintained their own airway throughout the procedure. This type of anesthesia is called:

   A) General anesthesia

   B) Conscious sedation

   C) Monitored anesthesia care

   D) Moderate sedation

35) For a spinal block for a one-time injection, where is the medication typically placed?

   A) The medication is injected into the subarachnoid space between L3 and L4.

   B) The medication is injected into the epidural space between L4 and L5.

   C) The medication is injected into the subarachnoid space between L1 and L2.

   D) The medication is injected into the subdural space between L3 and L4.

36) You are assisting with a procedure with the anesthesiologist providing sedation. The patient is injected with IV propofol and immediately starts gasping in pain and stating their arm is "on fire". What may be happening?

   A) The patient is having an adverse reaction to the propofol. Stop infusing immediately.

   B) The patients IV has infiltrated. Stop the propofol infusion and start another IV.

   C) The patient has received an overdose of the propofol. Stop infusion immediately.

   D) Pain at IV site is a normal reaction to IV propofol.

37) Which of the following is a safe drug to give a patient with a history of malignant hyperthermia?

    A) Sevoflurane

    B) Halothane

    C) Propofol

    D) Succinylcholine

38) Which of the following is not a reversal agent for nondepolarizing neuromuscular blocking agents?

    A) Neostigmine

    B) Edrophonium

    C) Bupivacaine

    D) Sugammadex

39) If your patient received which of the following medications, would you include in your post op discharge teaching to use a backup birth control plan?

    A) Sugammadex

    B) Neostigmine

    C) Propofol

    D) Sevoflurane

40) Signs of malignant hyperthermia include:

    A) Metabolic alkalosis

    B) Increased carbon dioxide- CO_2

    C) Decrease in carbon dioxide- CO_2

    D) Bradycardia

41) Your 6-month-old patient is scheduled to have non emergent surgery at 1100. Your patients mother tells you she breast fed the patient at 0600 this morning. What is your response?

   A) Cancel the surgery.

   B) Move the surgery to 1400 so the patient will have been NPO for 8 hours.

   C) Move the surgery to 1200 so the patient will have been NPO for 6 hours.

   D) Warn the OR nurse the patient will be cranky and continue as planned.

42) You are reading the orders for you per-op patient and see IV antibiotics ordered. You know IV antibiotics need to be given when?

   A) After the start of surgery

   B) Within 10 minutes of surgery

   C) Within 60 minutes of surgery

   D) 2 hours before surgery.

43) You are told in report your patient received a reversal agent at 1200. When is the soonest recommended time to discharge your patient home?

   A) 1230

   B) 1300

   C) 1330

   D) 1400

44) Your patient is having a rotator cuff repair surgery. You expect what type of neve block to be given?

   A) Interscalene

   B) Bier

   C) Quadratus lumborum

   D) Spinal

45) Your patient is admitted to the recovery room after a scleral buckling procedure where a gas bubble was injected into the eye to provide retinal tamponade. You plan to educate the patient on the physician's orders but expect to include what in your post op teaching?

   A) Patient must lay flat on back until follow up appointment

   B) Patient must maintain a face down position until released by physician.

   C) Patient must lay on non-operative side

   D) There will be no special positioning required.

46) Which of the following is not an antiemetic?

   A) Ondansetron

   B) Ketamine

   C) Promethazine

   D) Compazine

47) Which of the following is true of autologous blood transfusions?

   A) Blood may be transfused to other patients if not needed for doner.

   B) Blood must be donated 24 hours prior to surgery

   C) Patients do not qualify if they have cardiac disease, infections or seizure disorders.

   D) Patients may qualify if they are between the ages of 5 and 70.

48) What is not true of Hetastarch- Hespan?

   A) It is expensive

   B) It is derived from corn starch

   C) Allergic responses are rare

   D) It is an artificial colloid

49) You patient is admitted to the pre- op area for an amputation of a foot. The patient has heard horror stories about surgeons cutting off the wrong limb. The patient used a sharpie and put the word yes on the operative foot and a no on the non-operative foot. What is your next action?

   A) The patient is allowed to mark their own surgical site. Continue the pre-op process.

   B) The charge nurse should be called to double check the correct site.

   C) The anesthesia provider can remark the site before surgery.

   D) The surgeon still needs to mark the site even if the patient has as well.

50) Your patient had a large blood loss in surgery and continues to bleed. A blood transfusion is ordered but the patient's blood type is not available. What should be transfused?

   A) O negative

   B) O positive

   C) AB negative

   D) AB positive

CPAN/CAPA Example Questions Answers and Rationales

1) D

    Visceral pain is said to be not localized, deep pain such as from intraabdominal organs. Injured nerve pain is called neuropathic or radicular. Sharp pain from muscles, skin or joints is called somatic, this pain is well localized. Pain from inflammation is nociceptive which encompasses visceral, somatic and neuropathic. If this pain lasts longer than 6 months, it is termed chronic.

2) A

    Flumazenil reverses benzodiazepines.

3) B

    When the patient's spinal level is at T 10, the patient can feel sensation at the umbilicus, not below.

4) D

    A thoracic paravertebral block would be common for a thoracotomy. Axillary and supraclavicular blocks are for upper limb surgery

5) C

    Neuromuscular blocking drugs paralyze skeletal muscle.

6) A

    Oxytocin- Pitocin, is given post-delivery to help increase uterine contractions. Oxybutynin is a bladder relaxant. Oxycontin and oxycodone are pain medications.

7) B

    B&O suppositories are given to help relieve pain associated with bladder spasm. This medication is given after urology procedures.

8) D

    Norco is an opioid. Nifedipine is an antihypertensive and calcium channel blocker. Romazicon is a GABA receptor antagonist.

9) D

    Digoxin is a cardiac glycoside. Amiodarone is a noncompetitive adrenoceptor antagonist. Metoprolol is a beta blocker.

10) C

    Cold blood can cause cardiac output to decrease, not increase.

11) A

A Whipple can also involve removal of the gallbladder, common bile duct, part of the duodenum. This would be called a pancreaticoduodenectomy.

12) B

The correct safe way to move a 100 KG patient from the OR bed to a stretcher is anesthesia at head who Tells the team when to move, one person on each side of patient and one person at the feet.

13) A

American Society of PeriAnesthesia Nurses (ASPAN), is responsible for defining and establishing the scope of PeriAnesthesia nursing. The ANA- American Association of Nurses, the National League of Nursing- NLN, do not. SCIP stands for Surgical Improvement Project.

14) D

Salvaged autologous blood is saved through a special process in the operating room and reinfused into the patient.

15) D

The patient is probably in PEA- pulseless electrical activity. Compressions need to be continued.

16) A

Magnesium is commonly given for torsade's de point. Potassium would only be given if the patient has hypokalemia. Calcium would be given for hypocalcemia. Sodium bicarb would be given for acidosis.

17) C

TURP syndrome is caused due to the large amount of irritant used during surgery. Hyponatremia can be caused by this.

18) A

Chest pain, sudden fever, tachycardia and hematuria are common S/S of a hemolytic transfusion reaction.

19) D

A MAP of 65 mmHg is needed for adequate tissue perfusion.

20) B

A fasciotomy is done to release pressure. Pressure in a muscle compartment can exceed capillary perfusion pressure and can cause permanent muscle damage in 4 to 8 hours.

21) A

ERCP- Endoscopic retrograde cholangiopancreatography, relieves bile duct obstruction. TIPS- Trans jugular intrahepatic portosystemic shunt- is a procedure for portal decompression or for bleeding caused by portal hypertension. A PEG is a feeding tube. ICP stand for intercranial pressure.

22) C

ASPAN standards state there must be at least 2 RN's, at least one proficient in PACU care in the phase one unit.

23) D

This patient is an ASA 4 due to his comorbidities.

24) C

Beneficence is being kind. Autonomy is allowing patients to make their own choices. Justice is being fair. Fidelity is loyalty. Veracity is being trustworthy.

25) A

Corneas will typically heal on their own in 24 to 72 hours after injury.

26) D

The landmark for T 10 is the umbilicus. L2-3 is the knee. C7-8 is the middle finger.

27) B

Laying the patient flat may increase ICP. Hyperventilating the patient may help to decrease the CO2 which can help lower ICP.

28) B

Both provide PEEP. CPAP is continuous, BiPap provides pressure on inspiration, low pressure on expiration.

29) A

The three late signs of increased intercranial pressure – Cushing's triad- are hypertension, bradycardia and bradypnea.

30) C

Computer charting is not a requirement in a PACU.

31) D

This condition indicates the patient may stay paralyzed for a longer period of time after receiving succinylcholine.

32) B

After one unit of PRBC's the hemoglobin is expected to rise 1 g/dL and the hematocrit to rise 3%. PRBC's is centrifuged blood with most of the plasma removed.

33) A

Laryngospasm also can cause paradoxical chest movement, hypoxia. Call anesthesia, suction and bag patient as needed. The patient may need to be reintubated. Bronchospasm causes expiratory wheezing, tachypnea, prolonged expirations, accessory muscle use. Croup causes hoarseness, barking cough. A PE causes decreased breath sounds, dyspnea, tachycardia, hemoptysis.

34) C

Monitored anesthesia care involves a deeper level of anesthesia using IV propofol, benzodiazepines and/or opioids. The patient can maintain their own airway. Conscious sedation and moderate sedation are interchangeable terms that involve pain control and a lighter anesthesia. An anesthesiologist may not be needed for moderate sedation. General anesthesia involves placement of an airway.

35) A

One-time injection spinal anesthesia is typically injected into the subarachnoid space between L3 and L4.

36) D

Pain at the IV site is a normal reaction to receiving propofol. Reassure the patient it is temporary.

37) C

Propofol is the only drug listed that is safe for a patient with a history of malignant hyperthermia.

38) C

Bupivacaine is a local anesthetic medication.

39) A

Women of childbearing age should be told to use a backup birth control method if she has received Sugammadex.

40) B

Increase in carbon dioxide is a sign of malignant hyperthermia.

41) D

Breast fed patients need to be NPO for 4 hours prior to surgery.

42) C

IV antibiotics should be given within 60 minutes of starting surgery.

43) D

It is recommended to monitor patients for 2 hours after a reversal drug is given.

44) A

Interscalene block is most commonly given for rotator cuff repair.

45) B

It is common in procedures that include a air or gas bubble in the eye to have the patient remain in a face down position to keep the bubble in place.

46) B

Ketamine is a dissociative anesthetic.

47) C

Patients may not donate blood for autologous transfusions if they have cardiac disease, infections or a seizure disorder. Patients need to be between the ages 12 and 75 to donate. It is recommended to donate at least 72 hours prior to transfusion. Blood may not be given to other patients.

48) A

Hetastarch is not expensive. All the other answers are correct.

49) D

The surgeon needs to mark the surgical site if there is a potential bilateral site such as the patient having 2 feet or 2 arms where there may be a mistake, or if the surgical site is not obvious.

50) A

O negative can be given to anyone with any blood type in an emergency.

Study Reminders

Use this section to remind yourself of topics you would like to have more information on

Topic:	Topic:	Topic:
Topic:	Topic:	Topic:
Topic:	Topic:	Topic:

CAPA/ CPAN Crossword Puzzle

Across:

1) A term indicating minimal sedation. Patient responds normally but coordination may be impaired. Patient is able to maintain own airway.
2) A type of block when surgery is to be performed on a lower extremity.
3) A pain block done on the eye.
4) A scale used to determine pressure sore risk.
5) An anesthetic that can cause hallucinations.
6) Part of the Aldrete scale. Can involve feeling for a pulse, checking skin color and auscultating sounds in the chest.
7) A medication given to reverse the effects of benzodiazepines.

Down:

1) A sign of a medical issue that has caused nerve damage. Drooping eye lid, decreased pupil size, decreased sweating. Can be caused by spinal cord injury or stroke. Can be a potential complication of nerve blocks.
2) A scale using faces to indicate a level of pain. Used often for children.
3) A nerve block for surgeries performed on lower extremities.
4) A measurement of amount of carbon dioxide in exhaled air. Seen as a waveform.
5) An oral pain medication often prescribed to patients after outpatient surgery.
6) A non-depolarizing neuromuscular blocker, muscle relaxant. Given with general anesthesia.
7) A score used to assess the patient's readiness to be discharged from the PACU.
8) A medication given to a patient suffering from malignant hyperthermia.

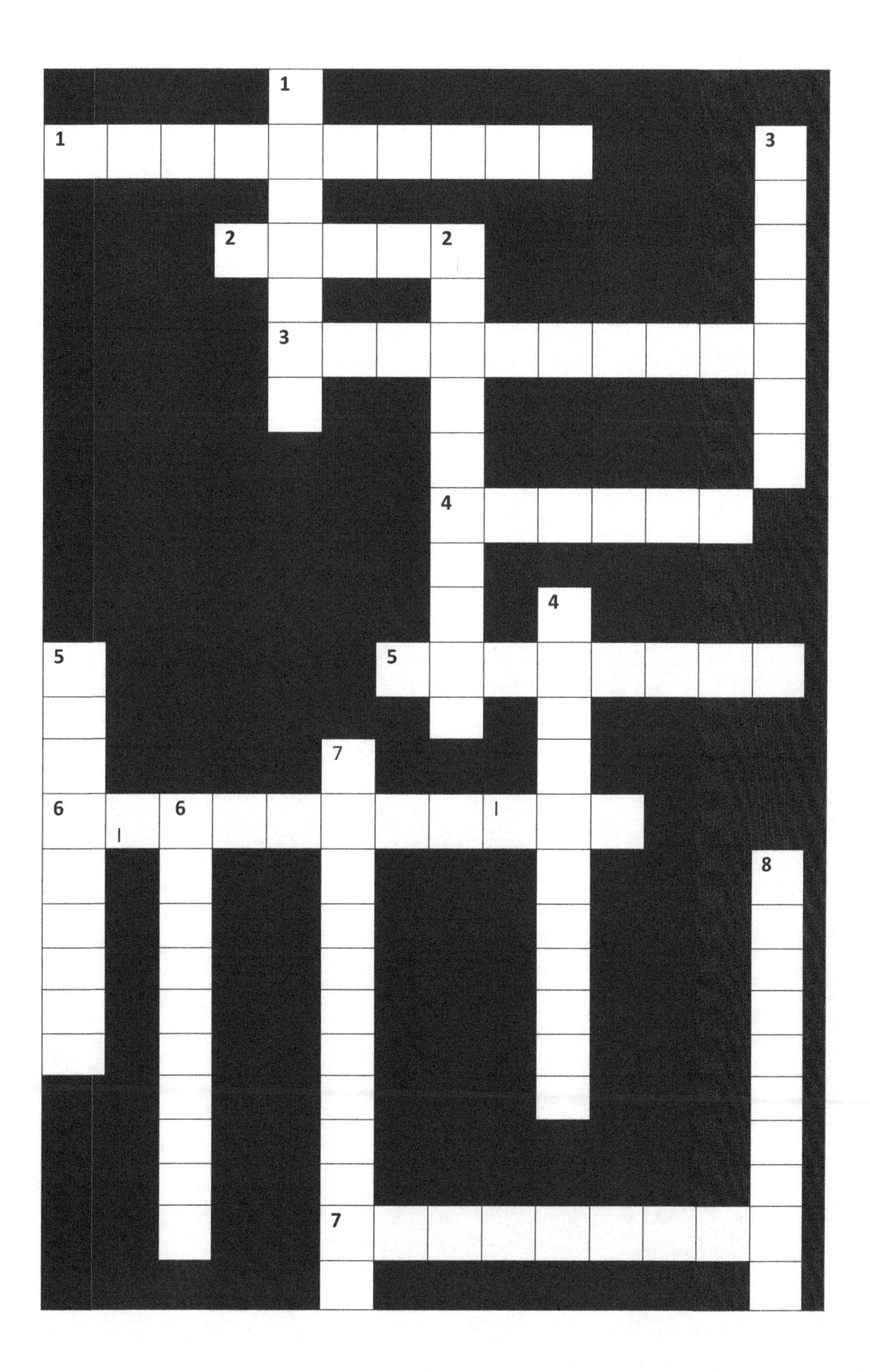

			1 H								**3** F
1 A	N	X	I	O	l	Y	s	I	s		E
			R								M
		2 A	N	k	I	**2** E					O
			E			w					R
		3 R	S	E	T	o	B	u	l	b	A
		S				N					L
						G					
						4 B	R	A	D	E	N
						A					
						k		**4** C			
5 O				**5** K	E	T	A	M	I	N	E
X				R				P			
Y			**7** A					N			
6 C	**6** I	R	C	U	L	A	T	I	O	N	
O	O		D					G			**8** D
D	C		R					R			A
O	U		E					A			N
N	R		T					P			T
E	O		E					H			R
	N		S					Y			O
	I		C								L
	U		O								E
	M		**7** R	O	M	A	Z	I	C	O	N
			E								E

84

Calendar

Sun	Mon	Tue	Wed	Thu	Fri	Sat

Calendar

Sun	Mon	Tue	Wed	Thu	Fri	Sat

Calendar

Sun	Mon	Tue	Wed	Thu	Fri	Sat

Calendar

Sun	Mon	Tue	Wed	Thu	Fri	Sat

Study Group Assignments

Name:	Assignment:

Blank Note Pages